# Relax
# Imagine
# Sleep

## with Help from Guided Imagery and the Soothing Sounds of Nature

from
WALKERCREST

Written and Illustrated by
Bryson Walker

# Walkercrest

ISBN: 9798863732947



First Printing October 2023

publishing@walkercrest.com

# DEDICATION

For Wayne, Joy, Jarrus, Jesica, Maia, Logan, Lylah, Megan and Davin. For your inspiration Leslie, may you always get a good night's sleep.

**IMAGINE** you have retired to your bedroom for the night.

Ah, night. The best time of day. Not that you didn't have good experiences while the sun yet shined. But you are satisfied with your efforts, with the service you gave others. And now, you are free of the demands found during daylight hours.

What is it about the hours beyond the sun's reach that makes you feel so free? You recall a poem by Walt Whitman that sums it up best.

> This is thy hour O Soul, thy free flight into the wordless,
> Away from books, away from art, the day erased, the lesson done,
> Thee fully forth emerging, silent gazing, pondering the themes thou lovest best.
> Night, sleep, and the stars.

You can hardly wait to rest your head on the downy pillow and let fade your place in society.

But first, why not crack open the window and let a little fresh air come in?

As you open the curtains you are thrilled to find a full moon and effervescent stars filling the late sky.

Now the moment is perfect. If ever there was a setting that could produce magical dreams it was this one. And you abandon yourself to the allure, fully succumbing to what will be the best and most enchanted night's rest of your life.

Ah, sleep, come quickly.

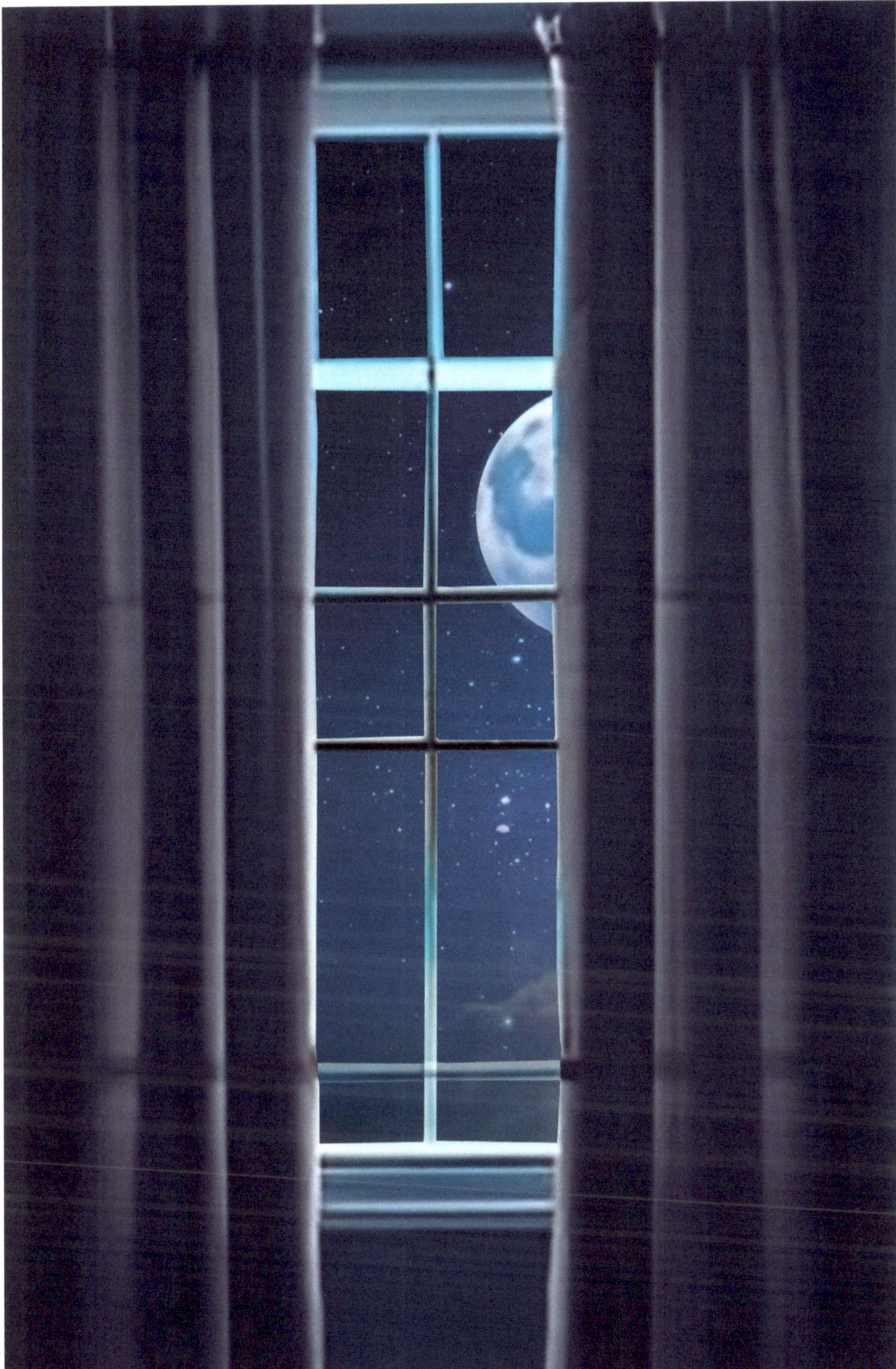

**IMAGINE** you will make a new friend in the form of a bird.

While it is common to bond with one's pet, in tonight's trip to a highland park you will develop an almost supernatural friendship.

You have been contemplating how you have not felt free to share the innermost feelings of your heart. Still, there is really nothing wrong with living a private life, is there? Then, as if on cue, an answer comes from within a rose tree. The soft chirping of a bird.

You decide to find out if it is talking to you. Could it be the "secret bird" of which the poet wrote? You recite the poem aloud.

I hid my heart in a nest of roses,
out of the sun's way, hidden apart:
In a softer bed than the soft white snow's is.
Under the roses I hid my heart.
Why would it sleep not? Why should it start,
When never a leaf of the rose-tree stirred?
What made sleep flutter his wings and part?
Only the song of a secret bird.

In the world of dreams I have chosen my part.
To sleep for a season and hear no word.
Of true love's truth or of light love's art
Only the song of a secret bird.

You wait for a response from the rose tree. But there is nothing. "Ah, well," you say out loud. "It's silly I suppose. What was I expecting in response to human words?"

Then you hear from the rose tree a chirp that fits perfectly the cadence.

"Only the song of a secret bird."

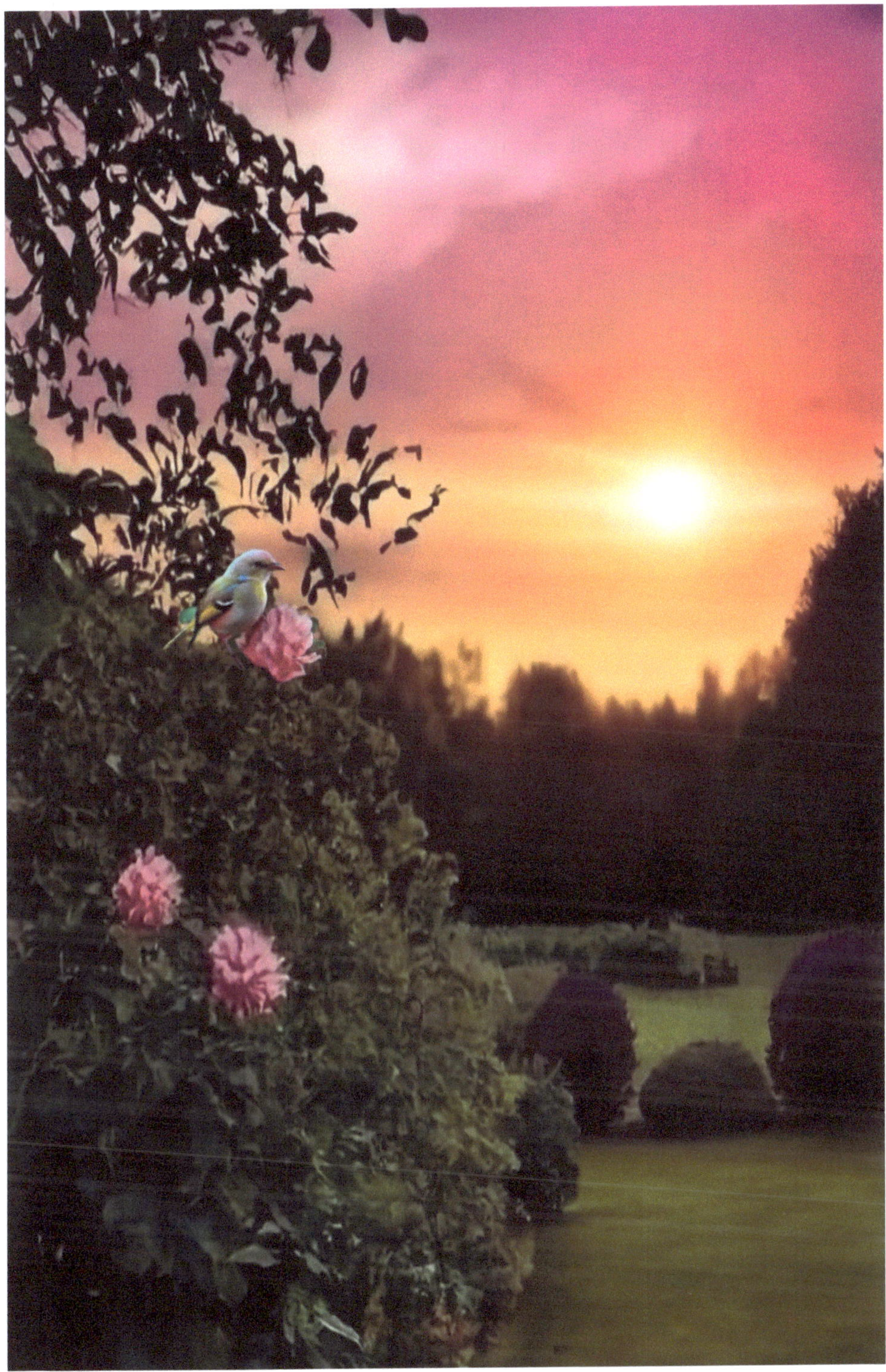

**IMAGINE** that you have inherited a bed and breakfast inn.

You have spent another long day fixing it up and now it is finally ready for guests. Tonight you feel different. Every other night, you returned home. But now, you wonder, "What would it be like to be a guest and actually stay overnight?"

You unconsciously make your way to the master suite. The room is beautiful with a bed you have been told is a rare antique. The thick mattress however is new and you laugh at yourself for feeling reluctant to try it out.

Moving to the window, it is as if you, a guest now, are seeing the backyard for the first time. There, a short distance from the patio is your favorite feature, an enchanting, natural waterfall. You listen to the cascading water and consider how wonderful this setting is. You almost wonder if you deserve to be here. And should you really sleep in this room tonight? You recall the poem you found hanging on a wall in the entryway. At first you took it down, but then decided to put it back up.

There is toil and there is test. And long the day but now recessed.
For nature's haven hath bequest, the fox its den, the bird its nest.
The day fulfilled, a time to rest. And be at peace, you did your best.

Emotions come to the surface as you think of the last line. You have to admit, "I really have done my best."

With the sounds of the waterfall soothing your tired mind, you surrender to nature and agree to treat yourself to a good night's sleep.

The bed is even more comfortable than you had imagined. A feeling of fulfillment overcomes you. You never really give yourself credit, but the truth is you really have done a lot. A lot of work. A lot of good.

The musical sounds of the waterfall seem to coax you into letting all your cares wash away.

You did your best, you deserve to rest.

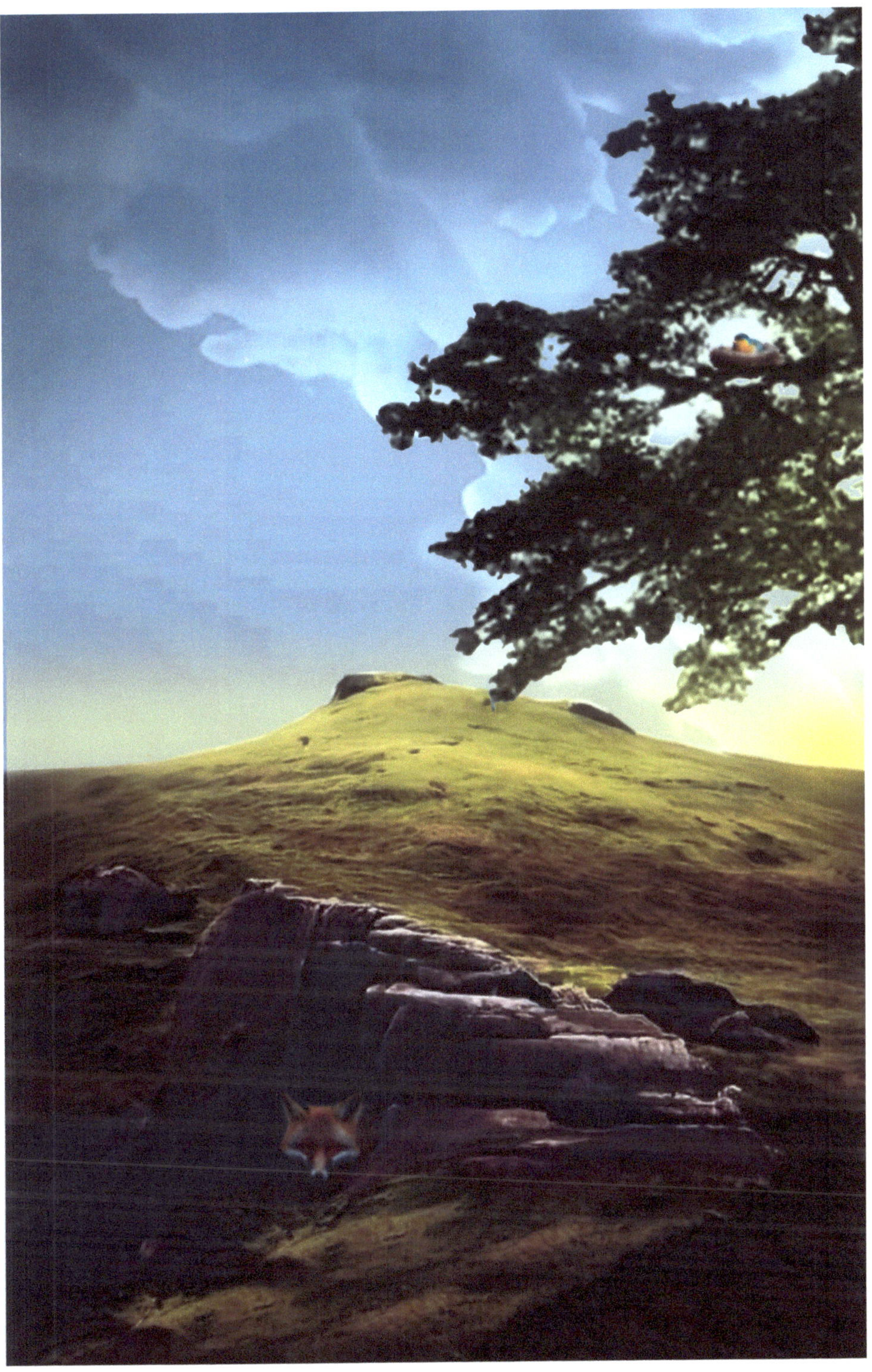

**IMAGINE** you have traveled to a little-known, uninhabited island.

Why have you been drawn here? Could it be that you are the descendant of sailing immigrants that once landed here?  Are their spirits whispering to you to find long lost buried treasure?

You explore. Circumnavigating the island you feel as though you have spent the day with those who came here long centuries ago.  And in fact that is the only treasure to be gained. But in some ways it is a treasure just feeling closeness to the past.

What would it have been like to be one of those early explorers?  You think of a poem by Longfellow.

Not enjoyment, and not sorrow is our destined end or way;
But to act, that each tomorrow find us farther than today.

Lives of great men all remind us we can make our lives sublime,
And, departing, leave behind us footprints on the sands of time;

Footprints, that perhaps another sailing o'er life's solemn main,
A forlorn and shipwrecked brother seeing shall take heart again.

Now you have returned to your own ship as the sun is setting. You climb aboard and give one last look to the island and its sandy shore.  You see your footsteps where you first set off to the north and where they come back from the south.  In the grand scheme of life there are many such circles.

Now a breeze fills your sails.

You wave farewell to this island like you have done so many times before, or so it feels.

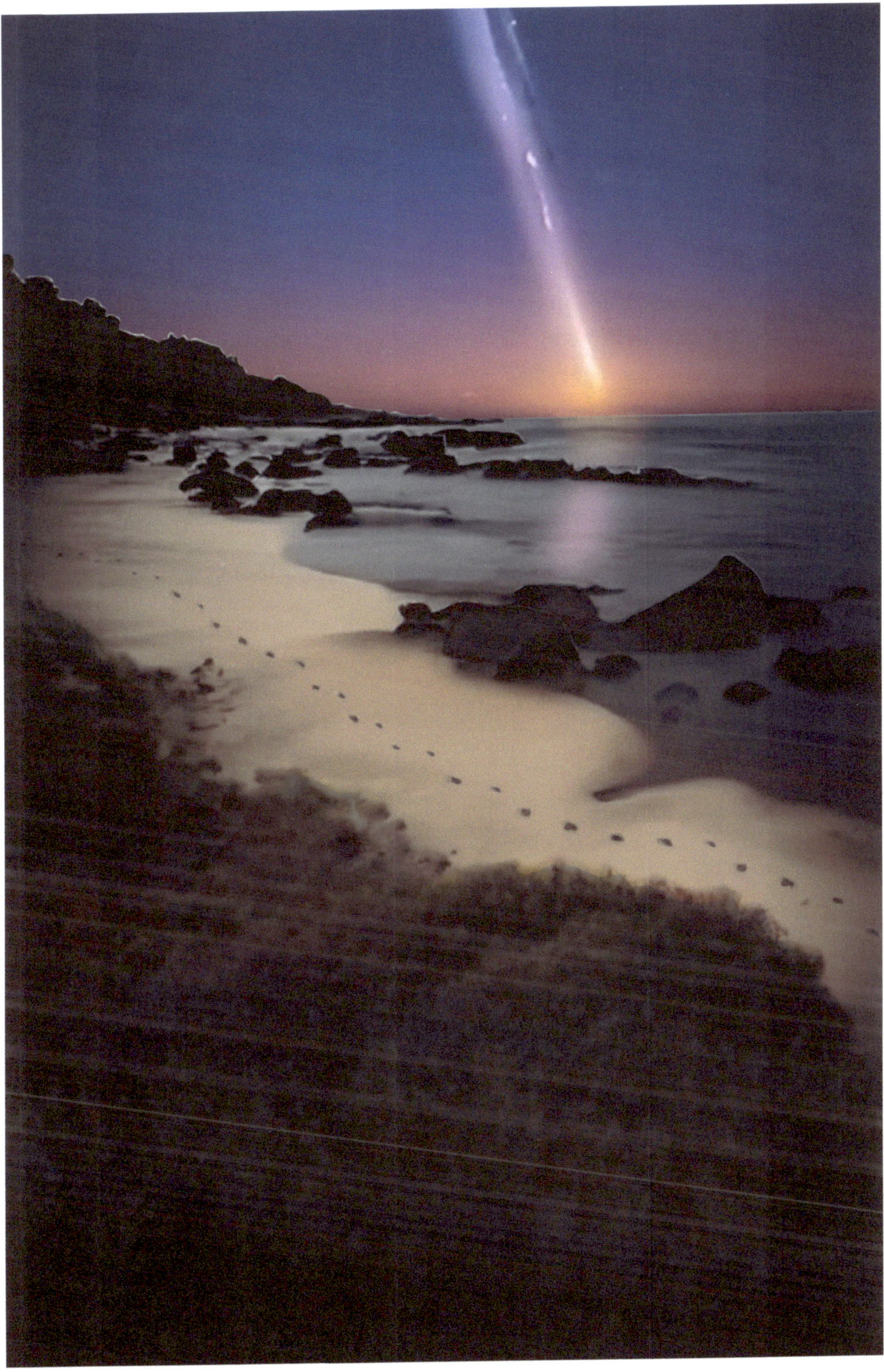

**IMAGINE** you are sailing back from the new world called America.

You have been months at sea on a grand voyage.

The lookout calls out from the crow's nest above, "Land ho!" You look over the rails in the twilight and see a vague outline on the horizon.

Could those be the coastal mountains of your home?

Next, a few lights on the shore become visible. Some of the sailors already in port will begin drinking and making merry in the taverns, but you, you are content to just be back within view.

Yes, you recognize it well now. That is indeed your port. Your quest has been successful and you have returned.

Homesick no longer, you recall this poem:

"Then let us sail on wings of angels,
May God guide us where-ere we roam.
The sea will grant each man new hope,
And in his sleep bring dreams of home."

Indeed, now you will sleep, and sleep well, because your dreams of reaching home are fulfilled.

You hear the dropping of the anchor. The plan must be to lay off the coast for tonight. That suits you. Let dawn wait. And with it will come a welcome of familiar faces and affection. For now, your work is over and you can relax. You pull a blanket around you and lie down.

With eyes closed you hear a sound that refreshes your very soul. A sound you had nearly forgotten. Peaceful oceans waves breathe up and down, in and out on the pebbled beaches of home.

Comfortable, content and deeply relaxed, you are serenaded by these sounds of the shore.

You thank the divine magic made where the sea meets the land, for it helps you fall into a deep, refreshing sleep.

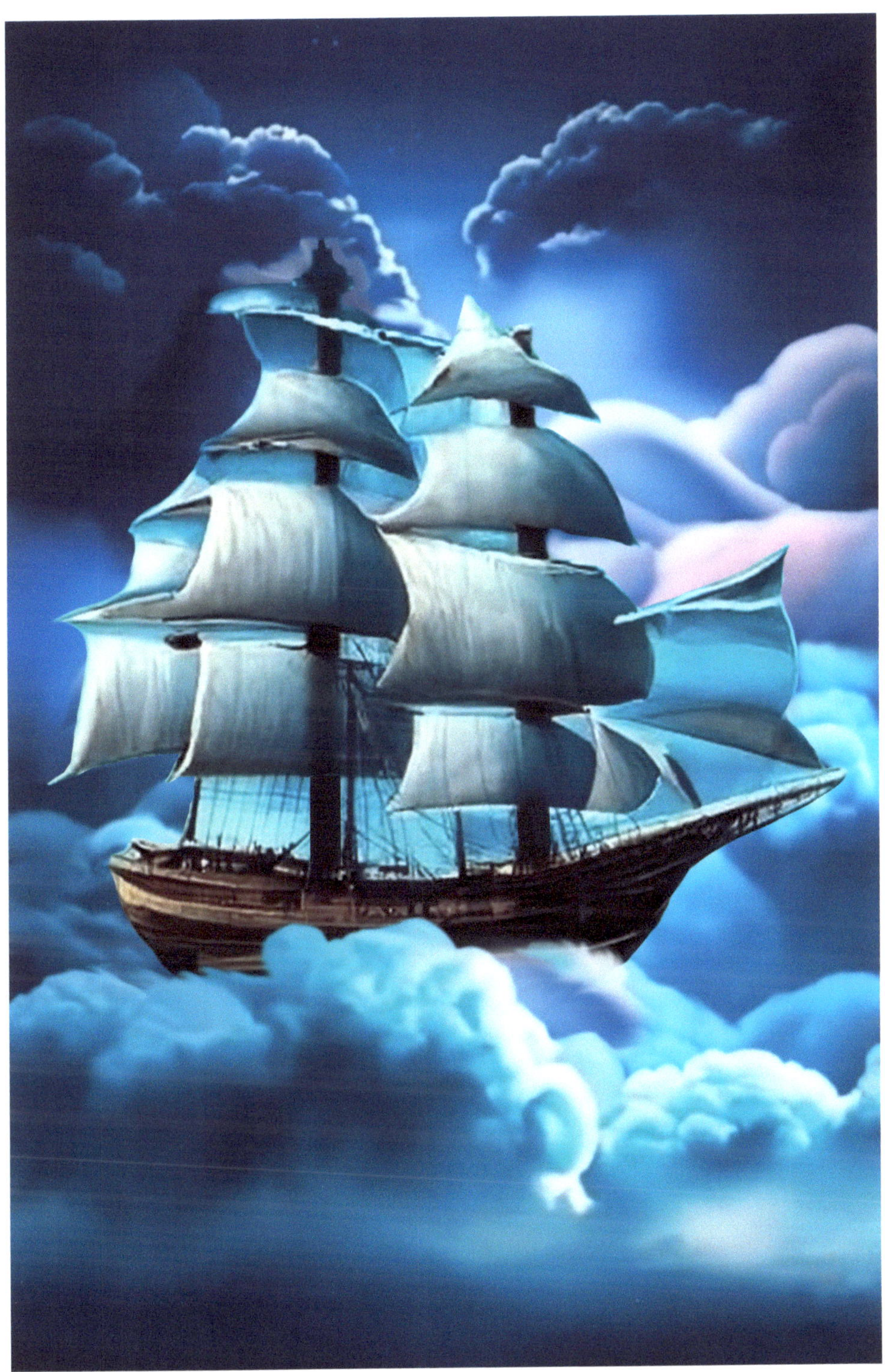

**IMAGINE** you are soaring above a mountain sea.

Alone in solitude, you feel as if your only companion is the soul of nature itself.

You recall a poem that seems to explain the oneness you feel with your surroundings.

The steadfast coursing of the stars.
The waves that ripple to the shore.
The vigorous trees which year by year
Spread upwards more and more.

The jewel forming in the mine,
The snow that falls so soft and light,
The rising and the setting sun,
The growing shade of night.

All natural things both live and move
In natural peace that is to say
To Him Whose strength sustains the world,
"Give us Thy Peace, we pray!"

Yes, the poet Parkes knows of where she speaks, for the scene you hover above is transcendant and otherworldy, yet, perfect to influence the dreams that you will soon entertain.

You return home and soon light upon your bed and pillow to drift into slumber where even more splendor awaits in your dreams.

You smile inwardly in thinking that a new dream will soon surpass even the glorious reverie of the mountain sea.

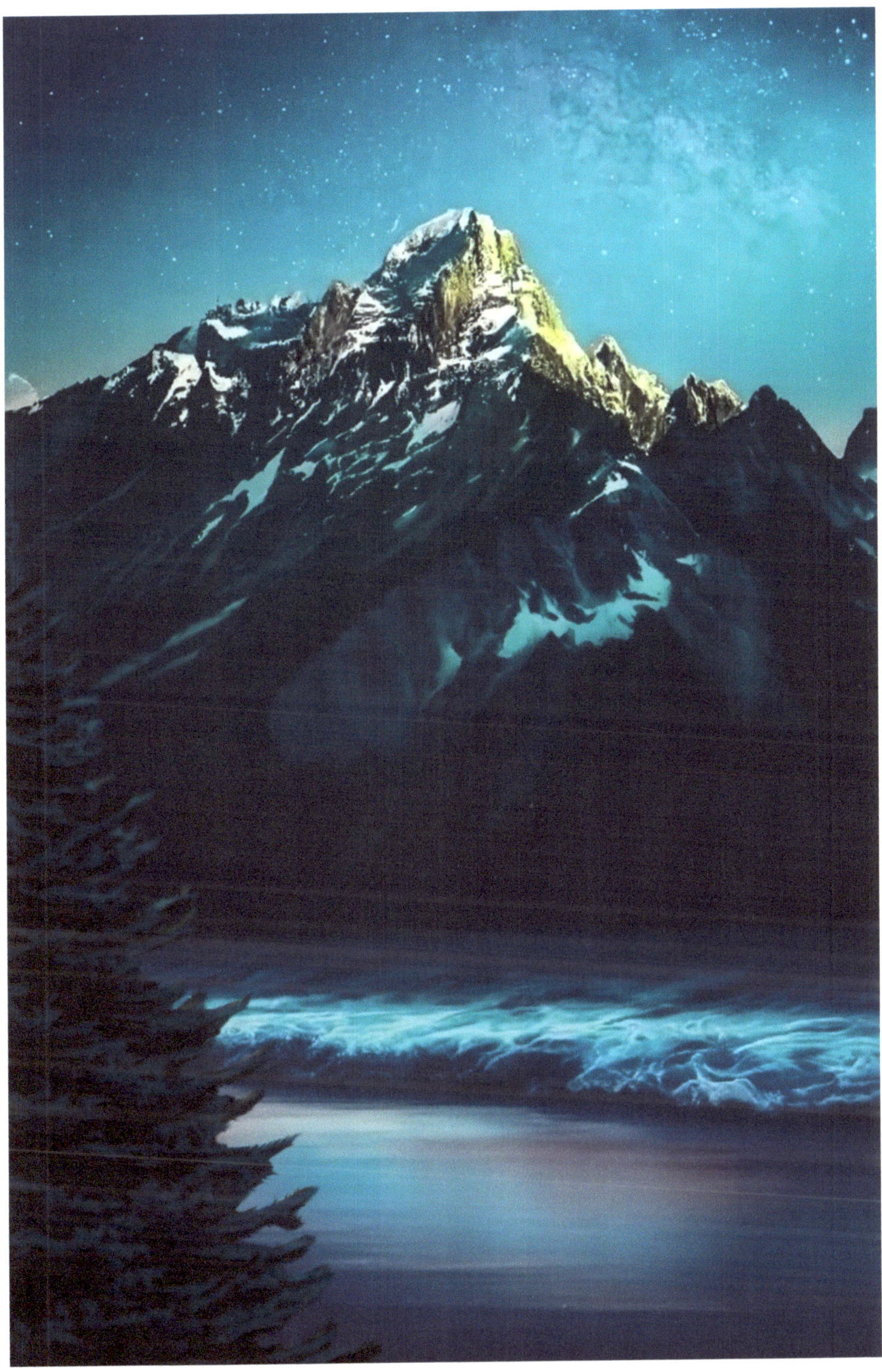

**IMAGINE** you are taking a nature walk on a forest path at sunset.

The waning sun gives the woods a yellow tint.

You are concerned that it is getting late and you don't want to get lost in the dark.

Looking ahead, you see you are coming to a fork in the road.

You stop to look far down the two paths, one to the left and one to the right.

Your view stops at the point where they bend behind the undergrowth.

You wish you could travel down both paths.

As night is falling, you decide with a sigh to take the one less traveled by.

Walking again, you are fortunate to find you have circled back to your cabin.

The last rays of sunlight give the logs a golden hue, quite pleasant-looking.

A melodic mountain stream runs behind, not far from the back porch.

Once inside, night falls quickly. The temperature outside begins to drop so you climb into your comfortable bed and reflect upon your good fortune.

You did not get lost.

You took the path less traveled and that made all the difference.

With eyes closed you listen to the calming stream outside your window.

A deep feeling of contentment and satisfaction comes over you.

The calming sound of the stream is nature's lullaby to help you relax and fall asleep.

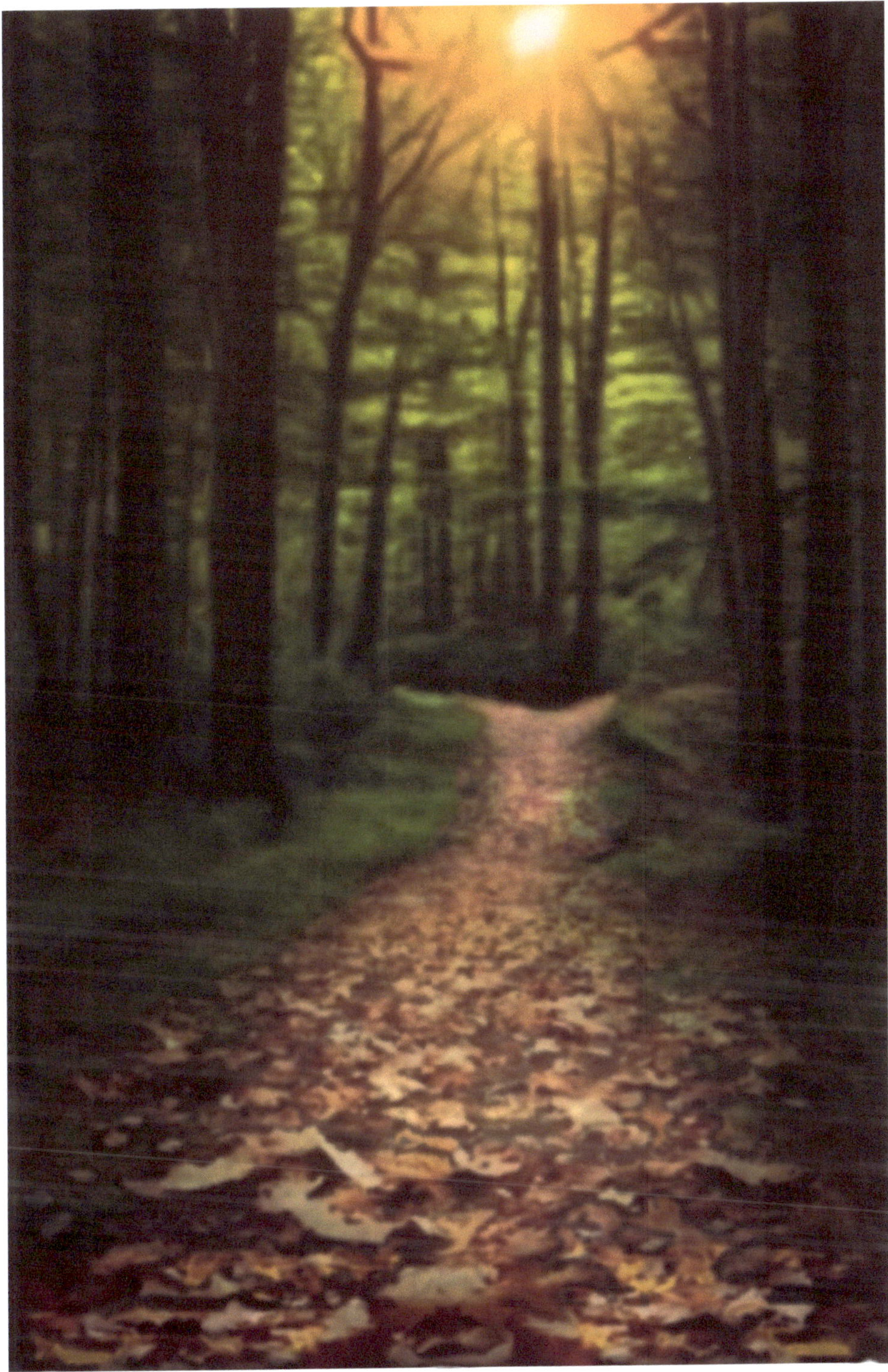

**IMAGINE** you are riding a horse on a snowy evening in 1922.

You are on a New England country road that takes you through some backwoods.

Night has fallen and the woods are dark and deep, yet beautiful in the moonlight.

After stopping for a short time to admire the scene, your horse shakes its harness bells to remind you there are still miles to go before you sleep.

Reluctantly you start off, leaving the woods and coming to a familiar lake.

The lights of your farmhouse reflect on the frozen ice.

Soon you are passing the farmhouse on the shore and you come to your own stables.

After brushing down your horse and giving it some oats you finally enter your own home.

You take off your coat and build a small fire in the wood-burning stove. It's good to be home. You have done and seen many things today.

Now, your tired yet fulfilled soul is soothed by the sounds of the cozy fire and the light wind outside.

Finally you allow yourself to relax, to lie down in bed.

You traveled miles before you could sleep.

And now it's time to go to sleep.

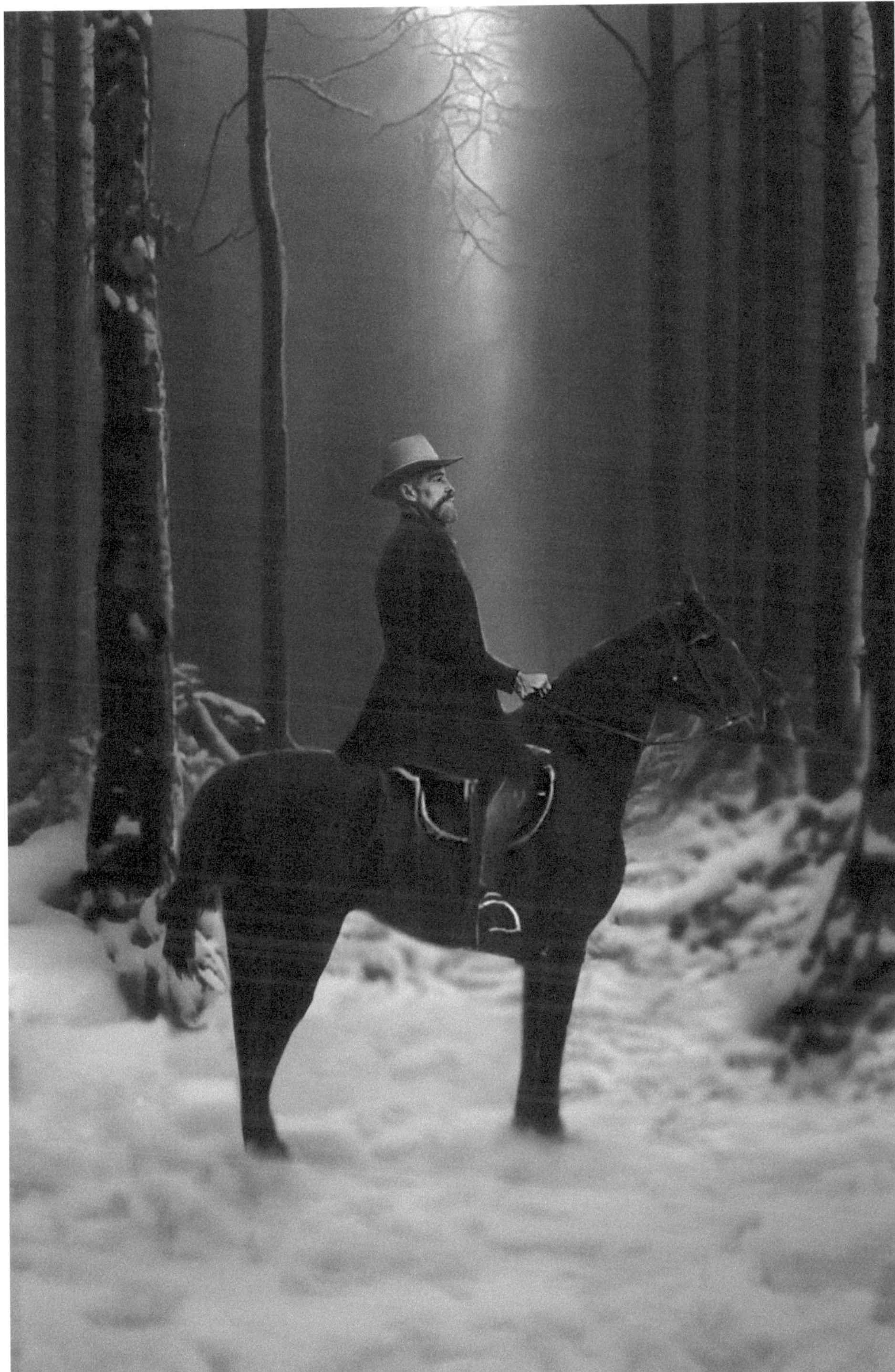

**IMAGINE** you have been given a royal garden.

Before today you were an average citizen, then came the news, you are the lost heir to a fiefdom.  They show you the deed and then the grounds of your inheritance.

First, a key in a black lock on an ancient iron gate, and then a dark green hedge, and then... a magnificent garden!

Would you like to take a tour?  "Yes," you reply. "But self-guided."

They protest. You insist.

"One moment for me please, and then I will share this with everyone."

As you walk into your garden, the words of the poet come alive in the voice of your mind.

There is another sky, ever serene and fair,
And there is another sunshine, though it be darkness there;
Never mind faded forests. Never mind silent fields.
Here is a little forest, whose leaf is ever green.
Here is a brighter garden, where not a frost has been;
In its unfading flowers I hear the bright bee hum:
Prithee, my brother, into my garden come!

"How well Dickinson's words fit this day," you think. "And how many people, like myself, have never experienced the beauty of such a place? It is mine to wrest away from the rich and share with all."

Maybe you imagine it, or maybe it is real, the garden seems to smile back at you, glowing with radiance.  Was there not a certain harmony between Robin and his Sherwood Forest?

The garden will be set free, as will the emotions of the people who visit. Tonight you will sleep as if rusty chains have dropped from your soul.

And sleep is necessary, for, with the garden, a new dawn is coming.

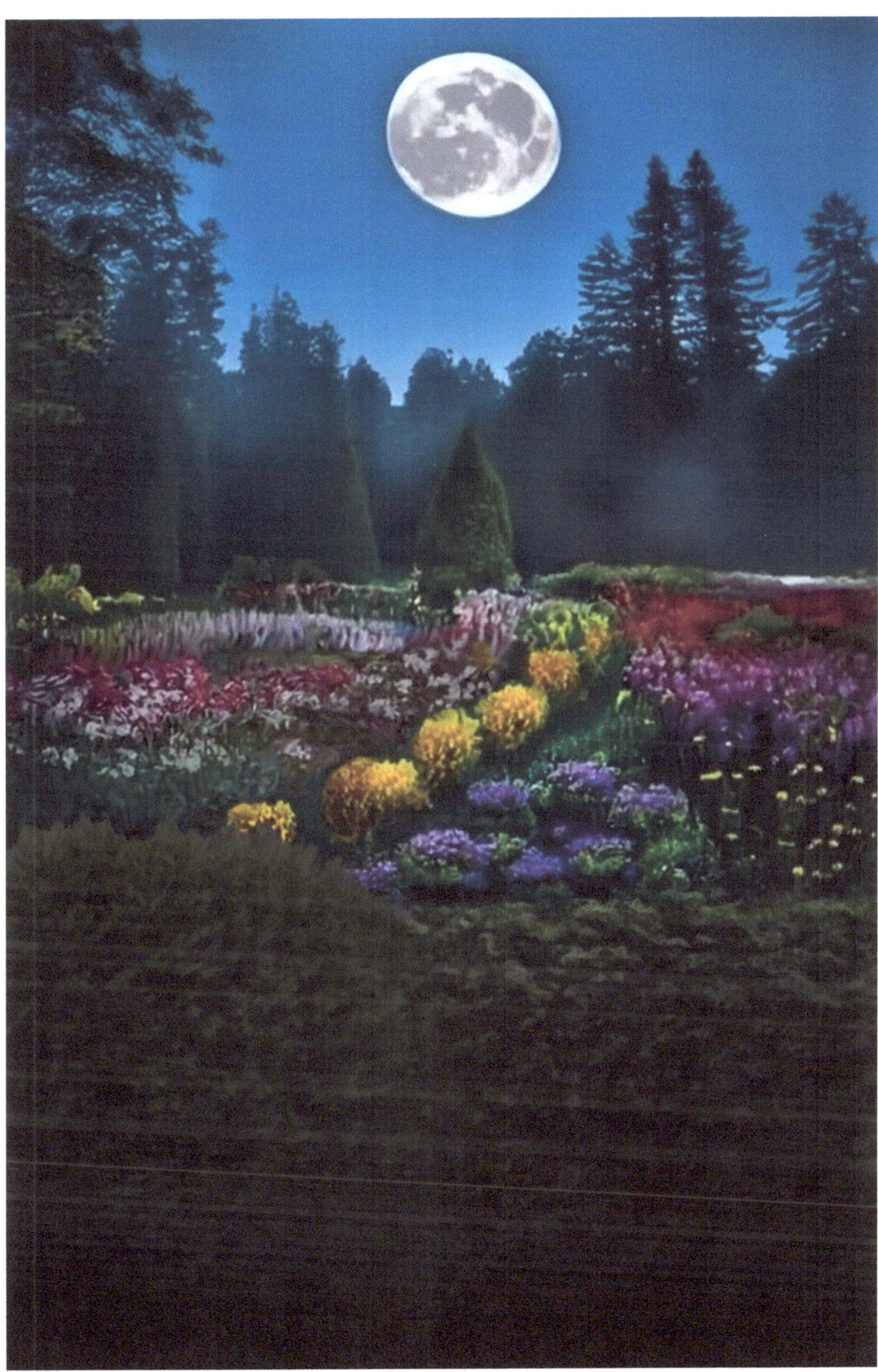

**IMAGINE** a mystic trail has taken your feet into the mountains.

Not knowing the way home, you sing Lead Kindly Light.

A peaceful wonder captures your imagination and you realize the earth is granting you an insight into her soul.

Words form in your mind, taking over the melody and you find yourself reciting:

Pray to what earth doth this sweet cold belong?
Wherein the moon glides up her cheerful path
In some far stratum of the sky?
By the brooksides, in this still, genial night
I, the more adventurous wanderer do hear
The sounds of gentlest summer means.

Is this verse from a poem by Thoreau?

Yes, and it transpired that he himself walked this same path long years past.

But did he traverse fair Walden Pond in the same manner?

For you float across it as if the water were fairy-touched and turned into enchanted ice.

At last the mystic trail takes your feet home. Soon you find you have fallen into bed unaware.

And without conscious effort a relaxation comes upon you, bringing forgetfulness to the fantasy, replacing it with sounds of the nighttime nature of the mortal woods.

From the mystic trail you have returned, returned to settle in the bliss of sleep.

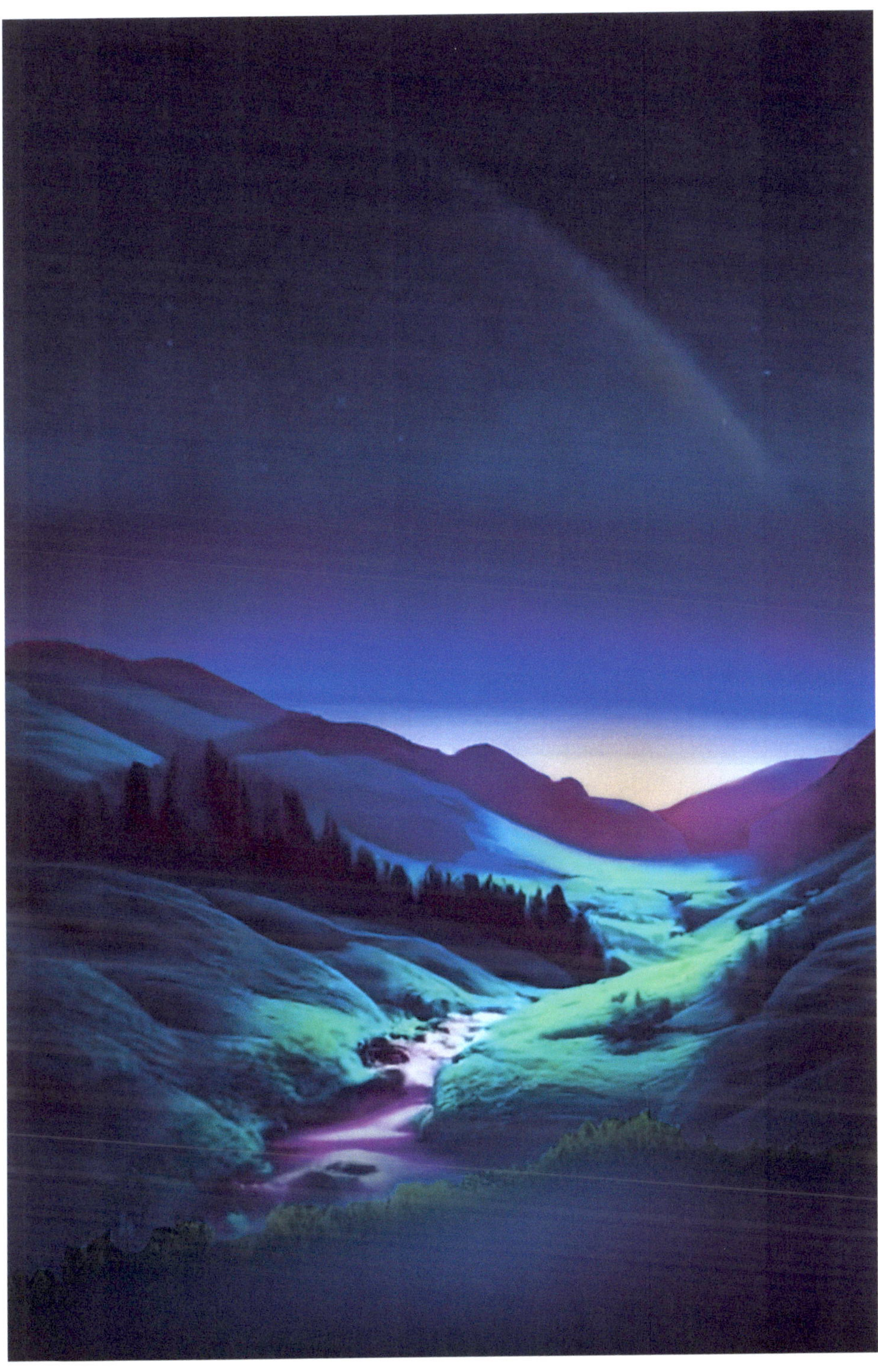

**IMAGINE** you have discovered a wild apple tree.

You have journeyed to the farmland of your ancestors.  Here and there are some remnants of days long past.  Your grandfather, or even his, may have partaken from this very tree.

You pick an apple and examine it.  Wiping it off on your shirt you consider taking a bite, but first a trick of the light makes you believe you see something in the polished reflection.  An autumn scene was there for a moment.  Simpler days as penned by the poet John Keats.

Season of mists and mellow fruitfulness,
Close bosom-friend of the maturing sun;
Conspiring with him how to load and bless
With fruit the vines that round the thatch-eves run
Where are the songs of spring? Ay, Where are they?
Think not of them, thou hast thy music too,
While barred clouds bloom the soft-dying day,
And touch the stubble-plains with rosy hue;
And full-grown lambs loud bleat from hilly bourn;
Hedge-crickets sing; and now with treble soft
The red-breast whistles from a garden-croft;
And gathering swallows twitter in the skies.

The poem persuades you that autumn is the best season of the year. Treasuring the apple, you take it with you on the return journey home.

Tonight, in the privacy of your room, you will hold it up in the window when the sunset dims and ask for autumn's enchanting reflection one more time.

And if your wish is granted, you will lie down and dream of your new favorite season.

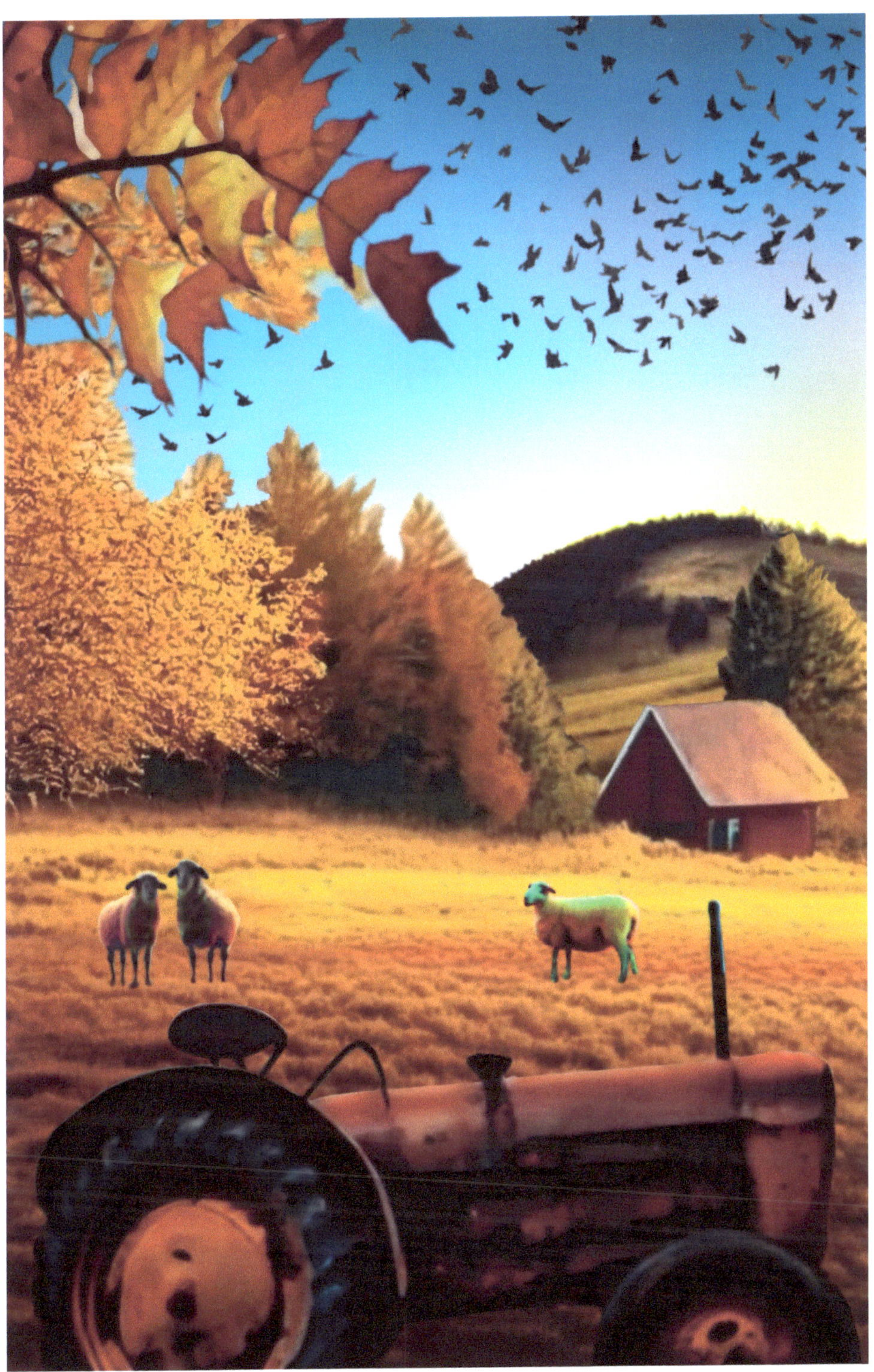

**IMAGINE** you are looking out the window of your castle.

In your mountain setting, the sun is quietly disappearing beyond the far horizon.  You have had a busy day and the start of night causes you to yawn.  Thinking of retiring, a poem comes to mind:

When sun falls heavy in the sky,
Bequeathing shadows from its eye
All bustle fails the more to try
To stay surrender as goodbye.
The creator's gold is sinking deep,
The curtain drawn by mountain steep
And calmer now that we must keep
The promise soon to beckon sleep.

Yes, sleep beckons.  Before you turn from the window however, you see a few drops of water splatter on the windowsill.  Well, that is good.  Let the sun shine during the day and let it rain at night.  The peaceful sound of rain will help drown out the thoughts in your mind.

Soon you are lying down and assume a comfortable position.  There is no need to resist sleeping, for as the poet said, it is time to surrender.

You close your eyes and listen as the rain has become steady.

You know this rain.  It is the long rain that comes with this land and it is a refreshing sound that will last all night.

How grateful and blessed you feel.  The added sound of rain has made the night perfect for drifting off in peace.

Yes, sleep beckons... and you are content to accept its call.

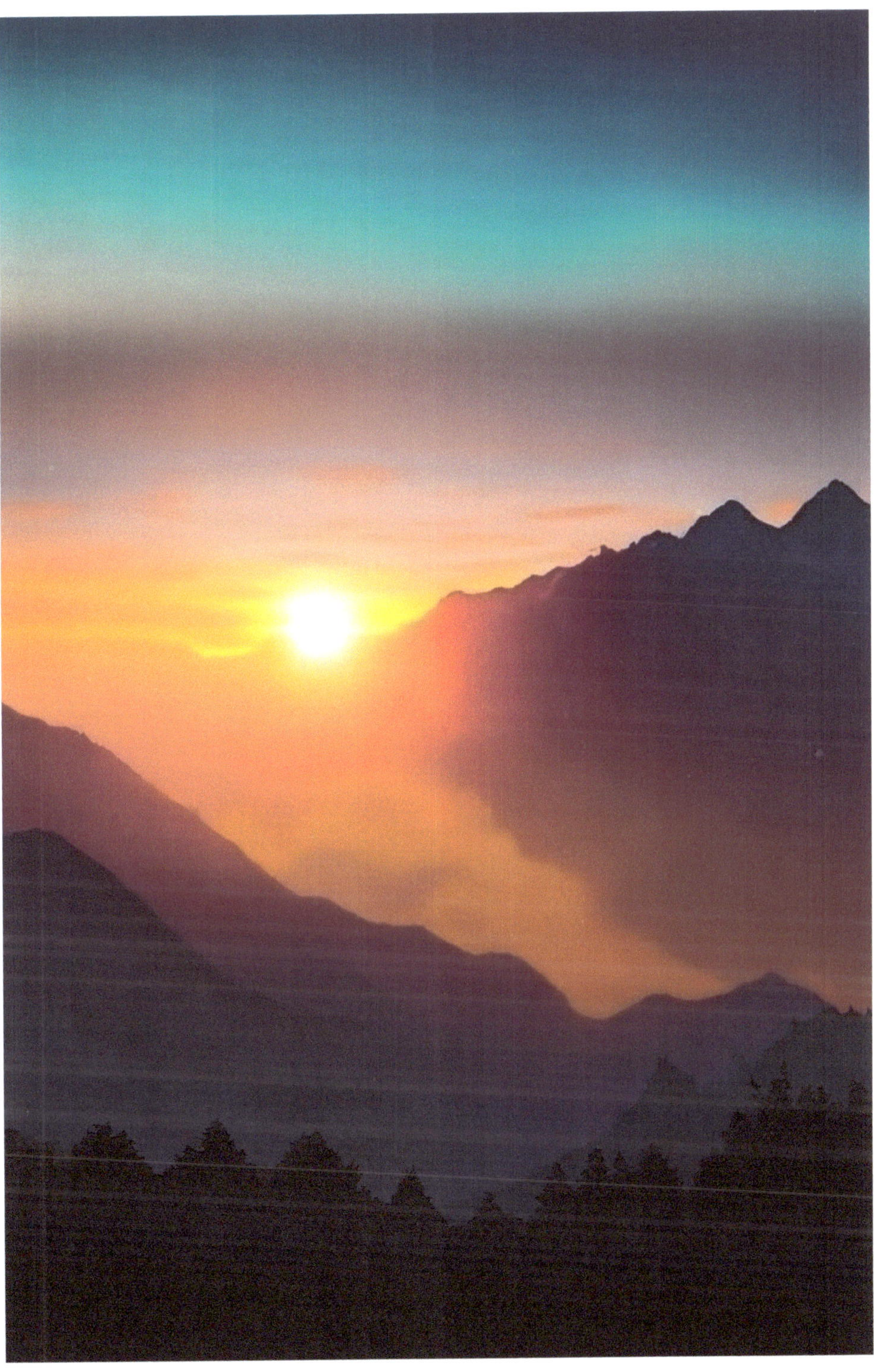

**IMAGINE** you are hunting mushrooms in forgotten Oregon woods.

Some may think your hobby is peculiar, but you dine on exotic flavors they have never before tasted.

Just in front of you, isn't that a black morel?  Bending down for a closer look you see instead a piece of wood.  Interesting. It is polished and rounded. A piece of a wagon wheel? What is it doing here?

Looking around, you feel as though you are playing the part of an actor from a poem written by Rudyard Kipling.

They shut the road through the woods seventy years ago.
Weather and rain have undone it again and now you would never know
There was once a path through the woods

Yet, if you enter the woods of a summer evening late,
When the night-air cools on the trout-filled pools
Where the otter whistles his mate
They fear not men in the woods because they see so few
The misty solitudes as though they perfectly knew
The old lost road through the woods

You have an urge to squint your eyes and cock your head a little.

Then, not in the direction you are looking, but more in your periphery you see–or rather you sense–the road taken by near-starving pioneers.

Why you feel a reverence for this place you can't say for certain. But rather than taking the remnant of history, you kneel back down and bury it in the earth.  When you return home you will also kneel down at your bed.

Perhaps it will make sense to no one, but you feel a kinship to that forgotten road and those forgotten trailblazers.  You will express thanks for the experience– for feeling an emotion quite unlike any other. And as you fall asleep there will come an answer, a resolution to this strange sense of longing, of melancholy, of veneration.

Thus enlightened, you will fall asleep, a changed person.

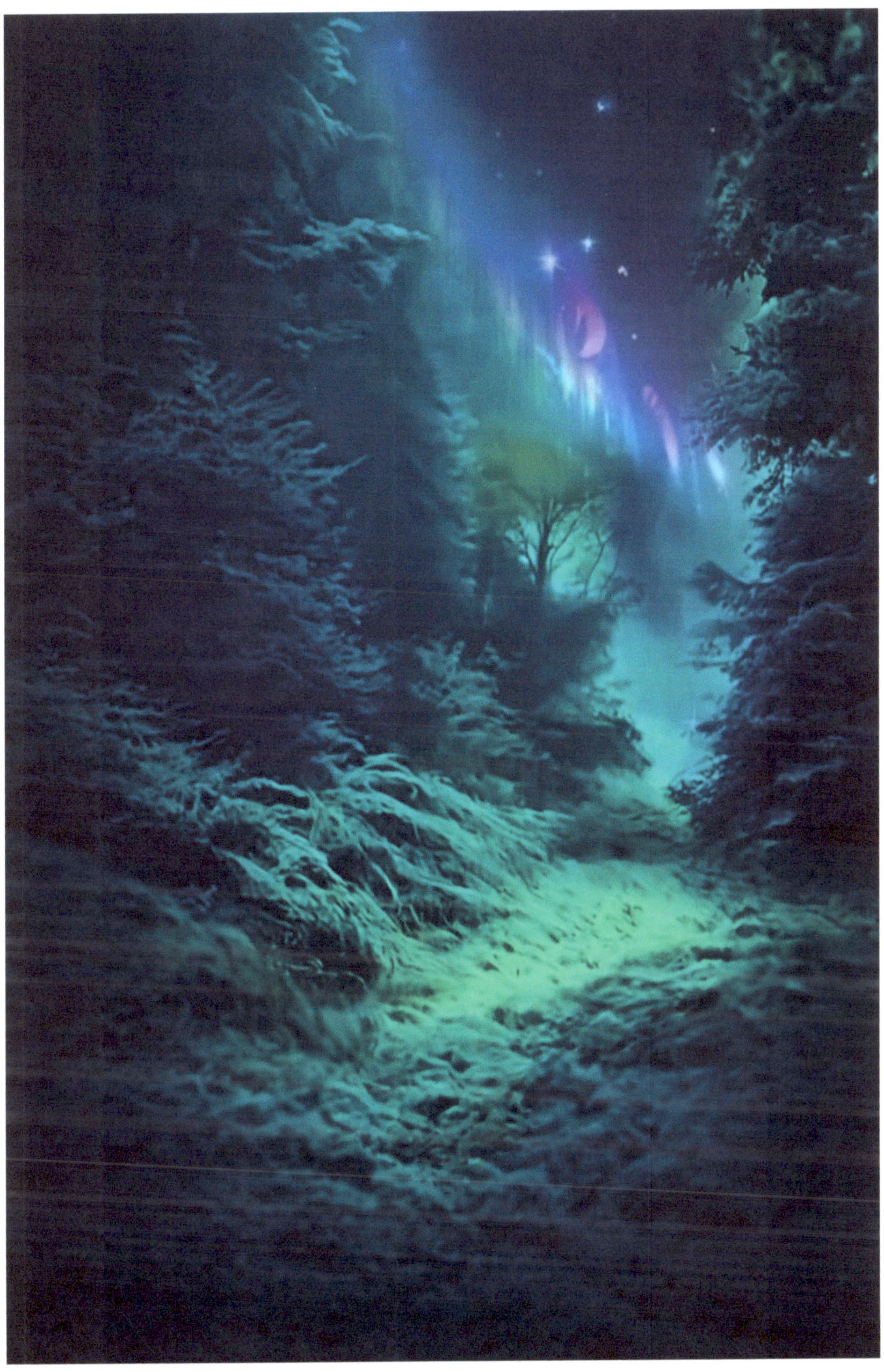

**IMAGINE** you have learned the silent secret of sleep.

It is so simple, yet you have not realized until this very night that the secret to falling asleep is to love the opportunity to dream more than reviewing the events of your life.

And why do you so willingly relinquish control of your mind to your imagination?

The poet may have said it best.

I love the silent hour of night,
For blissful dreams may then arise,
Revealing to my charmed sight
What may not bless my waking eyes.

Yes, centuries ago, Anne Brontë new the silent secret to sleep.

It is to love the opportunity to dream more than reviewing the events of your life.

And you acknowledge now that the day has come to an end.

The time is right to forget the cares of the world.

And to dream.

It is the silent secret of sleep.

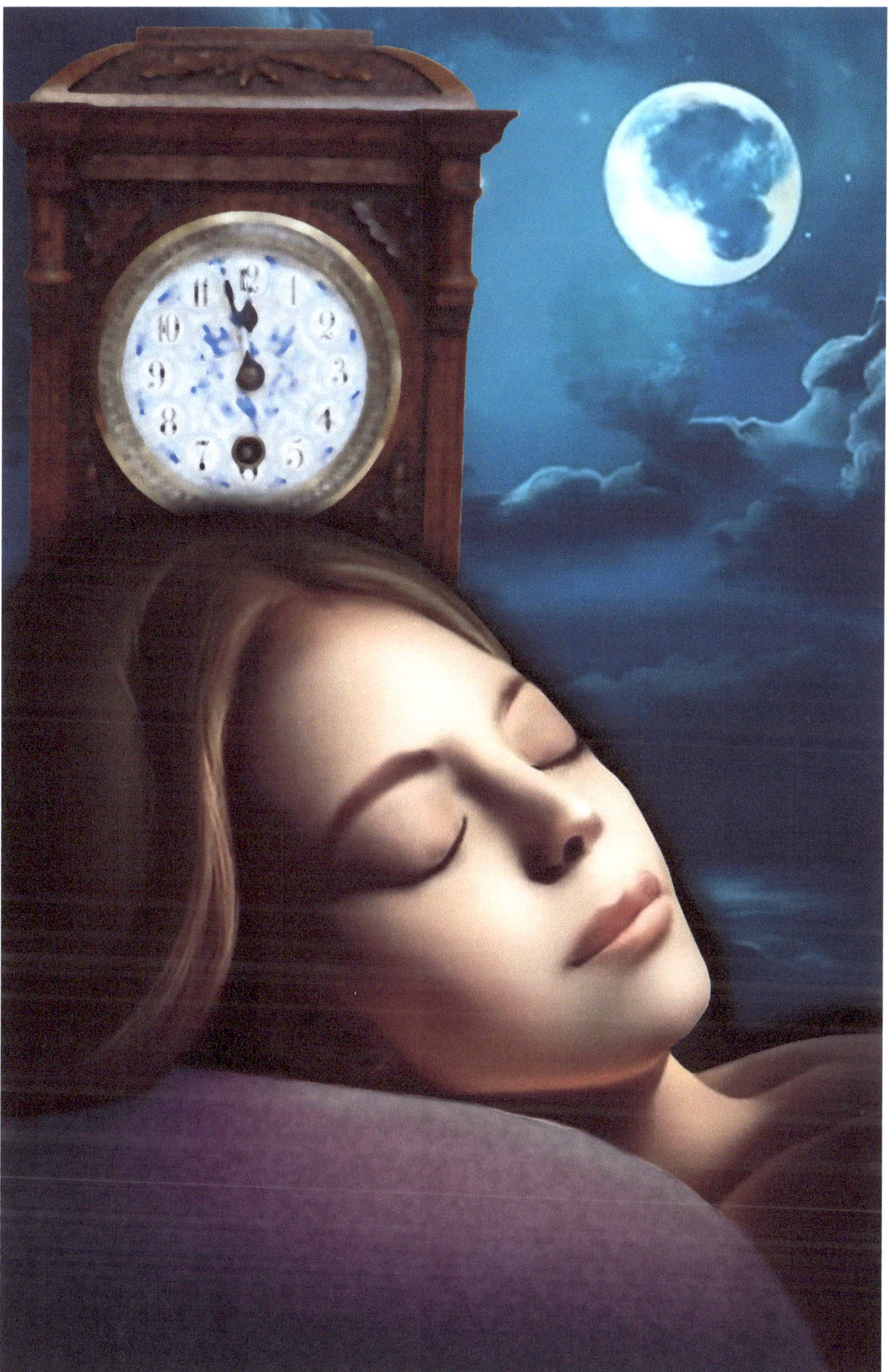

# About the Author and Artist

Bryson Walker studied art in college and has worked in many forms of media. The inspiration for this book actually came from his interest in audio programs that help people fall asleep.  "I personally like the sound of ocean waves, but I found that most of the surf sound effects were not peaceful.  I experimented with recording at different coastal locations until I found a beach where waves recede over pebbles. To me that was a similar sound to breathing in and breathing out."

Bryson had also produced a guided imagery audio program for a psychologist.  "Although his voice helped listeners fall asleep, I began experimenting with sounds of nature," Bryson explains. "The sounds of waterfalls and ocean waves seem to universally calm us."

Having collected sounds and poetry and recorded the audiobook, Bryson then began work on the art.  "I have friends that are excellent professional artists.  They gave me some tips on how to use my humble skills to create the illustrations for the book.  Remember, the printed book only exists because the audio proved effective first."

Bryson hopes people will have success relaxing and falling asleep with help from his efforts and the soothing sounds of nature.

Thank you for your patronage.

May you find other enriching titles available from Walkercrest

Please send any comments or suggestions to:

publishing@walkercrest.com